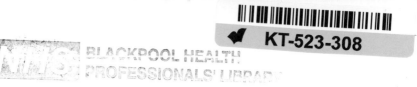
Presented as a service to medicine by

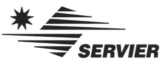

SERVIER

Prescribing information can be found at the back of the book

Biographies

Christopher J. Bulpitt qualified in Medicine at the University of London, UK, in 1963. He obtained his MRCP in 1967 and a MSc in medical statistics with distinction in 1972. In 1972 he was appointed senior Research Fellow at the London School of Hygiene and Tropical Medicine (LSHTM) and Honorary Consultant Physician at the Hammersmith Hospital and in 1974 Senior Lecturer in Epidemiology at LSHTM and then Senior Lecturer in Clinical Pharmacology at the Royal Postgraduate Medical School. His MD was awarded in 1975 and FRCP in 1982. In 1986 he was appointed a Reader in Pharmaco-epidemiology at LSHTM and subsequently, in 1987 he was appointed as a Reader in Epidemiology at the Royal Postgraduate Medical School. In 1989 he was awarded FFPM (by distinction) and became Professor of Geriatric Medicine at the Royal Postgraduate Medical School, now Imperial College School of Medicine. He has published over 400 scientific papers and has written/edited books on randomized controlled trials and hypertension. He was a member of the European Working Party on High Blood Pressure in the Elderly (EWPHE) and chairs the Data Monitoring Committee for the Systolic Hypertension in Europe trial (Syst-Eur). He is the lead investigator of the Hypertension in the Very Elderly Trial (HYVET) and his other current research interests include dementia, quality of life and the assessment of biological age.

Chakravarthi Rajkumar qualified in Medicine at the Madras Medical College in 1982. In 1986 he moved to Australia to take up a post of Research Fellow in cardiology at the Hallstorm Institute of Cardiology in Sydney. In 1994 he was awarded a postgraduate Medical Research Scholarship by the National Health and Medical Research council of Australia and worked at the Baker Medical Research Institute in Melbourne on cardiovascular adaptation with aging. In 1997 he was appointed as a Senior Registrar in Geriatrics at the Hammersmith Hospital and in 1999 was appointed as a Senior Lecturer in the Department of Medicine at the Imperial College School of Medicine. His current research interests include hypertension in the elderly and arterial compliance.

Nigel S. Beckett qualified in Medicine from the University of Manchester, UK, in 1990. His early training was at various hospitals in the north west of England and obtained his MRCP in 1994. He was appointed as Registrar in Geriatrics and General Internal Medicine in 1994 training at Bolton and Manchester hospitals. In 1996 he was appointed as Senior Registrar in Geriatrics and General Internal Medicine working at the University Hospital of South Manchester. In 1998 he became a British Heart Foundation Research Fellow at Imperial College School of Medicine and is currently the co-ordinator of HYVET.

John Potter is Professor and Head of Division of the University Division of Medicine for the Elderly, University of Leicester, UK, and Head of the Acute Stroke Unit and Honorary Consultant Physician at The Glenfield Hospital, Leicester. His research interests cover three main fields: cerebrovascular disease, hypertension, and cardiovascular physiology in relation to aging.

Professor Potter is an Executive Member of the British Hypertension Society and Member of the British Hypertension Society Blood Pressure Guidelines Committee. He also serves on the Research Into Ageing Research and Development Committee and The Stroke Association Research and Development Committee.

CLINICIAN'S MANUAL

HYPERTENSION AND THE ELDERLY

C.J. Bulpitt

C. Rajkumar

N. Beckett

Division of Geriatric Medicine
Imperial College School of Medicine
Hammersmith Hospital

London, UK

Foreword written by J.F. Potter

SCIENCE PRESS

Published by Science Press Ltd, 34–42 Cleveland Street, London W1P 6LB, UK.

© 1999 Science Press Ltd.

http://current-science-group.com/

British Library Cataloguing in Publication Data.

A catalogue record for this book is available from the British Library.

ISBN 1-85873-301-4

This copy of *Clinician's Manual on Hypertension and the Elderly* is given as a service to medicine by Servier Research Group. Sponsorship of this copy does not imply the sponsor's agreement with the views expressed herein.

Although every effort has been made to ensure that drug doses and other information are presented accurately in this publication, the ultimate responsibility rests with the prescribing physician. Neither the publishers nor the authors can be held responsible for errors or for any consequences arising from the use of information contained herein. Any product mentioned in this publication should be used in accordance with the prescribing information prepared by the manufacturers. No claims or endorsements are made for any drug or compound at present under clinical investigation.

Project editor: Mark Knowles
Illustrator: Stuart Malloy
Typesetter: Simon Banister
Designer: Claire Huntley
Production: Adrienne Hanratty
Printed in the UK

Contents

Acknowledgements

Figure 1.1 Adapted with permission from Kannel WB. **Epidemiology of essential hypertension: The Framingham experience.** *Proc R Coll Phys* 1991, **21**: 273–287.

Figure 1.2 Adapted with permission from Kannel WB. **Epidemiology of essential hypertension: The Framingham experience.** *Proc R Coll Phys* 1991, **21**: 273–287, and from Swales JD (ed). *Manual of Hypertension.* Oxford: Blackwell Science; 1995.

Figures 1.3 and 1.5 Adapted with permission from Truswell AS, Kennelly BM, Hansen JDL, *et al.* **Blood pressure of !Kung bushmen in northern Botswana.** *Am Heart J* 1972, **84**: 5–12.

Figure 1.4 Adapted with permission from Bulpitt CJ, Fletcher AE. **Ageing, blood pressure and mortality.** *J Hypertens* 1992, **10** (suppl 7):s45–49.

Figure 2.1 Adapted with permission from Staessen J, Amery A, Fagard R. **Editorial review: Isolated systolic hypertension in the elderly.** *J Hypertens* 1990, 8:393–405.

Figures 3.1 and 3.2 Adapted with permission from Gueyffier F, Bulpitt CJ, Boissel J-P, *et al.* **Antihypertensive drugs in very old people: a subgroup meta-analysis of randomized controlled trials.** *Lancet* 1999, **353**:793–796.

Table 3.4 Adapted with permission from MRC Working Party. **Medical Research Council trial of treatment of hypertension in older adults: principal results.** *Br J Med* 1992, **304**:405–412.

Tables 3.5, 3.6, and 5.6 Adapted with permission from Bonapace S, Rajkumar C, Bulpitt CJ. **Tailoring anti-hypertensive treatment in the elderly.** *J Hum Hypertens* 1998, **12**:615–620.

Foreword

Coronary artery and cerebrovascular disease remain the major causes of death and disability in westernized societies in those over 65 years of age, with hypertension being the major treatable risk factor. We are also faced with increasing numbers of elderly people, particularly those who are 75–79 years of age, whose numbers have increased by over 40%, and those who are over 80 years of age, whose numbers have increased by nearly 60% in the past 30 years. However, the elderly have been a much-neglected section of the community in terms of research into cardiovascular disease, particularly hypertension, although matters have changed considerably during the past 10–20 years.

Hypertension is common among elderly people, and results in a significant increase in coronary artery and cerebrovascular disease. However, there are important differences between young and elderly patients with hypertension, and these differences cannot be neglected when considering assessment, investigation, and treatment. Many significant large intervention studies in both combined hypertension and isolated systolic hypertension in older people have been reported in the past few years. This has resulted in a general increase in enthusiasm for treating elderly patients with hypertension, particularly as the absolute benefits in terms of reduction in stroke and heart attack are greater than in younger age groups. The aims of this book are to provide general practitioners and hospital physicians alike with a comprehensive summary of the important physiological changes associated with hypertension in older people and to summarize the most appropriate investigations and treatment regimens based on recent trial work. It is hoped that this small, but in-depth synopsis will provide a useful guide to all those treating elderly patients with hypertension and go at least some way towards improving the health of older people.

J.F. Potter
June 1999

Introduction

'Hypertension is the most common treatable disorder of the aged. As the general population increases in age, it is an increasingly important public health concern.'[1]

In developed countries, blood pressure rises with age. Therefore, the proportion of elderly patients with blood pressure high enough to place them at risk and to warrant reduction exceeds that in the rest of the population. It also follows that most of the people with hypertension that are seen in general practice are classifiable as elderly (ie, over 65 years of age).

Most of the data from early clinical trials in hypertension are from middle-aged male patients. However, there are now enough trials of treatment of hypertension in the elderly to lay down guidelines and make decisions on the management of these patients.

This manual provides specific guidelines on the management of hypertension in elderly men and women, as the pathogenesis of their condition differs from that of hypertension in younger people. Hypertension in the elderly is more likely to be of the isolated systolic variety and the response to antihypertensive agents may differ from that in younger patients. Many elderly hypertensive patients have other diseases that will influence the choice of antihypertensive agent. The implementation of lifestyle changes to reduce blood pressure tends to become more difficult with advancing age. Presently, there is limited data on the benefits of treatment in those over 80 years of age. There is debate on whether hypertension in the very old should be treated at all.

The manual covers all of these points. It starts with the epidemiological evidence for the growing problem of hypertension in the elderly, describes briefly its pathophysiology, and reviews the randomized controlled trials of treatments exclusively in older patients. It describes the problems faced by the clinician in assessing and investigating hypertension in the elderly and covers its pharmacological and non-pharmacological management. It ends with an approach to the particular problems of elderly patients with hypertension, such as stroke, orthostatic hypotension, drug interactions, and concomitant diseases.

Hypertension is not a disease in itself, but is a risk factor for other diseases, such as coronary heart disease, stroke, and renal failure. It may be an isolated risk factor, or just one part of the cluster of insulin resistance and consequent hyperinsulinemia, hyperlipidemia, and glucose intolerance that has been described as the insulin resistance syndrome.[2] In the past, clinicians have often considered hypertension in the elderly to be a natural phenomenon of ageing and have left it untreated. This manual strongly promotes the message that this approach is a mistake. It is offered to general practitioners and hospital doctors as a concise guide to hypertension and its management in the elderly.

Epidemiology

Chapter 1

Epidemiology

Blood pressure in Europeans and North Americans increases with age throughout the duration of an individual's life, but tends to remain in a similar centile of the general population's pressure. If a baby has a blood pressure in the top 5% of the normal distribution at six weeks of age, it is likely to be in a high position after six years and to remain so in middle age. This blood pressure 'tracking' process also determines that the higher the initial blood pressure, the greater the rise in pressure later in life. Low birth weight and high placental weight are related to high blood pressure in middle age, suggesting that events in intra-uterine life help to determine it.[3]

However, the people with the highest blood pressure in middle age are not necessarily those with hypertension in old age. For those individuals in the upper centiles, hypertension begins to take its toll in middle age, with heart attacks, strokes, and heart failure leading to early death in those whose hypertension has not been controlled *(Figures 1.1 and 1.2)*. Therefore, the elderly patient with hypertension is a survivor, with perhaps different physical characteristics from the patient with hypertension who died when ten or twenty years younger.

Until about 50 years of age, systolic and diastolic pressures rise in parallel, and cardiovascular risk is linked to both. However, above this, age-associated arteriosclerosis progresses and reduced arterial compliance leads to a relatively lower diastolic pressure, so that the hypertension becomes more exclusively systolic *(Figure 1.3)*. In the very old, low diastolic pressure is associated with previous myocardial infarction, dementia, and

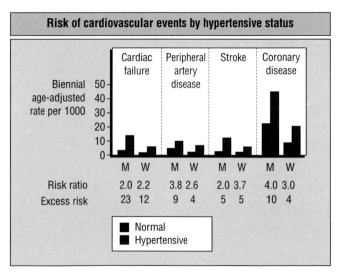

Figure 1.1 Data are from subjects of 35–64 years of age, after 36 years of the Framingham Study. M, men; W, women.

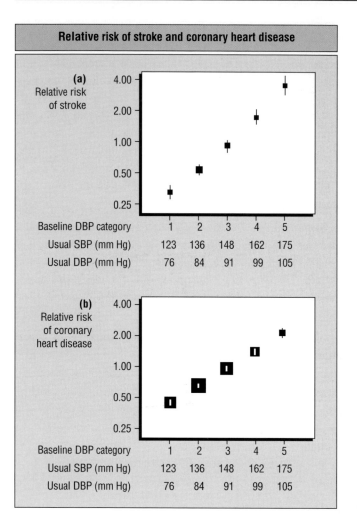

Relative risk of stroke and coronary heart disease

(a)
Relative risk of stroke

Baseline DBP category	1	2	3	4	5
Usual SBP (mm Hg)	123	136	148	162	175
Usual DBP (mm Hg)	76	84	91	99	105

(b)
Relative risk of coronary heart disease

Baseline DBP category	1	2	3	4	5
Usual SBP (mm Hg)	123	136	148	162	175
Usual DBP (mm Hg)	76	84	91	99	105

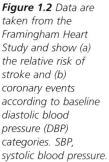

Figure 1.2 Data are taken from the Framingham Heart Study and show (a) the relative risk of stroke and (b) coronary events according to baseline diastolic blood pressure (DBP) categories. SBP, systolic blood pressure.

malignancy. It is suggested that very elderly patients with hypertension live longer than their peers with a 'normal' blood pressure do.[3]

Facing the risks

Fear that reducing blood pressure in the elderly may lead to an increase in deaths from coronary thrombosis has made many doctors reluctant to treat hypertension in these patients, especially as their low diastolic pressure may be linked with postural hypotension. Many believe that administering an antihypertensive drug to an older

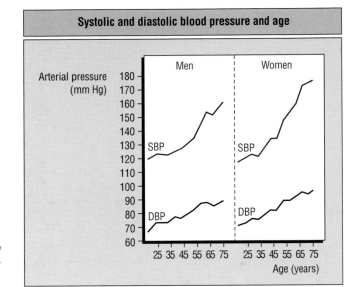

Systolic and diastolic blood pressure and age

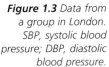

Figure 1.3 Data from a group in London. SBP, systolic blood pressure; DBP, diastolic blood pressure.

patient may worsen the postural hypotension and thus decrease the quality of life, even if theoretically it might reduce the risk of stroke.

However, the risk of stroke in the elderly is high. In developed societies, the 10-year risk of a major cardiovascular event in people with mild hypertension is < 1% in those who are 25–34 years of age and > 30% in those who are 65–74 years of age (*Figure 1.4*).[4] There is both experimental and clinical evidence that reducing hypertension in the latter group significantly reduces this risk.

Types of hypertension in the elderly

Isolated systolic hypertension (ISH) is defined as a sustained systolic blood pressure ≥ 160 mm Hg and a diastolic pressure ≤ 90–95 mm Hg.[5] Two major reviews have reported the prevalence of casual diastolic hypertension in the elderly to be 11–40%.[6,7] In the 1993 Health Survey for England, 41% of men and 40% of women over 75 years of age had a casual systolic blood pressure reading of ≥ 160 mm Hg.[8] These figures are supported by the finding that among those over 75 years of age in Britain, hypertension and heart failure together account for over half of all general practitioners' consultations.[9]

Such casual measurements of blood pressure in a cross-section of the population are useful. However, the measurement of sustained high blood pressure in prospect-

5

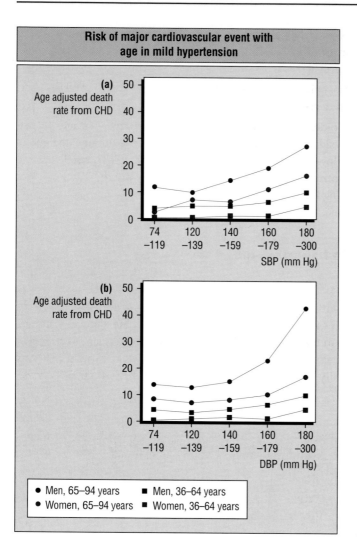

Risk of major cardiovascular event with age in mild hypertension

(a)

Age adjusted death rate from CHD

SBP (mm Hg)

(b)

Age adjusted death rate from CHD

DBP (mm Hg)

● Men, 65–94 years   ■ Men, 36–64 years
● Women, 65–94 years   ■ Women, 36–64 years

Figure 1.4 Data are from the Framingham Study at 30-year follow-up and show age-adjusted death rate from coronary heart disease (CHD) according to five ranges of systolic (SBP) and diastolic blood pressure (DBP).

ive surveys is more important in assessing the long-term burden of the disease. In the elderly population[10]:

- Sustained systolic hypertension affects 6–12% of people over 60 years of age, is higher in women, and increases with age.

- Sustained diastolic hypertension affects 12–14% of people over 60 years of age, is higher in men, and decreases with age.

- Sustained systolic plus diastolic hypertension affects 6–8% of people over 60 years of age, is higher in women, and increases with age.

- Sustained isolated systolic hypertension affects 1–3% of men of 60 years of age and 4–13% of women of 70 years of age. It is more common in women and increases sharply in prevalence with age.
- Sustained isolated diastolic hypertension affects 5–9% of people over 60 years of age, mostly men, and decreases with age.

The fact that so many older people have sustained hypertension, of whatever pattern, has given rise to the idea that it is almost physiological – the classical top end of the bell-shaped curve. However, this does not explain why people in rural communities in developing countries show no such rise with age *(Figure 1.5)*.[11] Factors other than age must be inducing the rise in the developed world.

Factors related to hypertension in the elderly

Salt

Studies of populations with different salt intakes and randomized, controlled trials of reduced salt intake suggest that differing sodium intakes alter blood pressure. However, they disagree in their estimate of the size of the effect. Analyses of pooled study results estimate that systolic/diastolic pressures rise by 4–5 mm Hg for every 100 mmol increase in daily sodium intake.[12,13] The effect of sodium on blood pres-

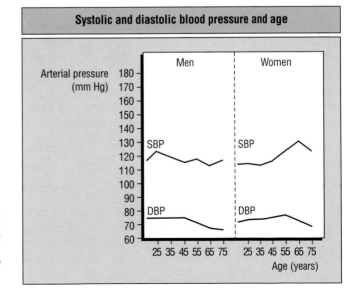

Figure 1.5 Data from a group of !Kung bushmen. SBP, systolic blood pressure; DBP, diastolic blood pressure.

sure increases with age: this may be because of the adverse effects of a lifetime's over-consumption of sodium, or because with advancing age it becomes more difficult to maintain a normal sodium balance.

Obesity

Body weight is closely and directly related to blood pressure at all ages. In INTER-SALT, for the same average height, a 10 kg difference in weight was associated with a 3 mm Hg difference in systolic pressure and a 2.2 mm Hg difference in diastolic pressure.[14] An adolescent's weight strongly predicts blood pressure later in life.

Physical exercise

Blood pressure is inversely related to physical exercise and physical fitness[15], although how closely they are related is yet to be elucidated. Study results are confounded by self-selection of fitter people into the high exercise groups and because different studies used different definitions of exercise. However, long-term follow-up of college graduates has shown that those who exercised vigorously throughout their lives were to some extent protected from developing hypertension in later life.[16]

A sedentary lifestyle may therefore be partly to blame for rising blood pressure – and most people become more sedentary as they grow older. This theory is supported by the finding that physical training reduces blood pressure. Changing to a high-energy-expending lifestyle causes systolic/diastolic pressures to fall by a mean of 10/8 mm Hg in patients with hypertension, by 6/7 mm Hg in those with borderline hypertension, and by 3/3 mm Hg in normotensive patients.[15]

Alcohol

There is a popular conception that a small amount of alcohol per day may reduce blood pressure and a larger amount increase it. However, the available data does not fully support this, and a direct relationship between the amount of alcohol consumed and blood pressure is confirmed in many studies.[17] J-shaped studies have been described, proposing that non-drinkers have a higher blood pressure than those drinking up to 2–3 drinks a day, but the fact that ex-problem drinkers may have been included in the teetotal group should be considered.

The largest study to date is the U.S. Kaiser Permanente Study of 80,000 men and women up to 79 years of age.[18] This did not have a J-shape; rather it concluded that systolic pressure increased by 1 mm Hg for each daily unit of alcohol. In another American study, the rise in blood pressure with alcohol intake increased with age, being higher in people from 50–74 years of age than in those of 35–49 years of age.[19] The type of alcohol consumed in these studies made no difference to the height of the pressure-raising effect, so it is assumed that ethanol is the direct cause.

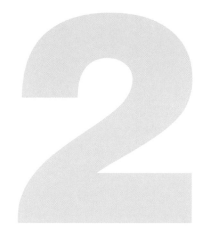

The pathophysiology of hypertension in the elderly

The pathophysiology of hypertension in the elderly

The pattern of the changes in systolic and diastolic pressures that occur with advancing age gives a clue to the pathophysiology of hypertension in the elderly. While diastolic pressure remains constant or declines after the age of 50 years, systolic pressure rises steeply from the age of 60 years onwards *(Figure 2.1)*.[20] In individuals who are 60–69 years of age, the prevalence of sustained systolic or diastolic hypertension is 8%, rising to a value of 22% in those over 80 years of age.

This increase in systolic pressure is explained by age-related stiffening of the walls of the large arteries. Large arteries are not simply passive tubes transporting blood from the heart to the periphery. In addition to conducting and distributing blood, they have endocrine and paracrine functions, and they buffer the pulse of the heart, smoothing out the flow of blood to the smaller arteries and beyond.

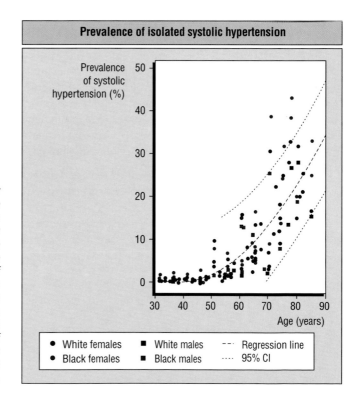

Figure 2.1 Data show the midpoint of the age classes reported in various studies. As shown by the regression line, the prevalence of systolic hypertension rises curvilinearly with age. The 95% confidence interval (CI) for the prediction of individual points is presented for the age range 50–90 years.

The main structural differences between the large and small arteries are in the media, which in the former is made up of elastic fibres and collagen fibres, and in the latter is muscular. The elastic fibres and collagen give the large arteries their capacity to dilate to accommodate the wide changes in flow and pressure generated by the beating heart. The smooth muscle in the smaller arterial wall produces the resistance that maintains mean arterial pressure.

In aging large arteries such as the aorta, arteriosclerosis leads to the replacement of the elastic fibres and collagen by fibrosis, so that its expansile properties are reduced. The large arteries become more rigid and therefore much less compliant, so that the pressure waves induced by the heartbeat are not dampened and travel at a greater velocity. Their transfer further along the arterial tree, plus reflection of pressure from the periphery in systole, results in systolic hypertension.[21]

This change is complicated by the fact that older patients with hypertension have lower renin levels and are more sensitive to sodium repletion than younger patients are.[22] The low renin levels suggest that the renin–angiotensin system is unlikely to be a cause of the hypertension. On the other hand, sympathetic control of the circulation does change with age. Vascular smooth muscle cells (as in the media of the smaller arteries) do not lose their alpha-adrenergic responsiveness with age[23], but age does dull the sensitivity of beta-adrenergic receptors.[24] This produces an imbalance in which the alpha-adrenoceptors stimulate vasoconstriction that is not opposed by vasodilating beta-receptor activity.

The effect of atheromatous change (which is more common and more extensive in older people) on the vascular endothelium also contributes to hypertension in the elderly. An endothelium denuded by atherosclerosis continues to produce vasoconstricting factors such as endothelin, thromboxane, and angiotensin II, but is no longer able to produce the vessel-relaxing factors nitric oxide and prostacyclin.[25] The result of this imbalance is a tendency towards rising peripheral resistance.

More than 90% of elderly hypertensives have essential (primary) hypertension. Most cases of secondary hypertension in this age group are drug-induced or have an underlying renal cause, while a small number are due to endocrine or neurological causes. *Table 2.1* lists the causes of secondary hypertension in the elderly. The rare condition of pseudohypertension occurs in an atherosclerotic brachial artery that is incompressible, and therefore gives a false high reading on the sphygmomanometer.

Causes of secondary hypertension in the elderly
Drugs
Corticosteroids
Estrogen replacement
Non-steroidal anti-inflammatory drugs
Alcohol
Ergotamine
Antihistamine/sympathomimetic decongestants
Liquorice
Renal
Renal artery stenosis
Pyelonephritis
Glomerulonephritis
Obstructive neuropathy
Analgesic nephropathy
Polycystic kidney disease
Connective tissue diseases
Endocrine
Conn's syndrome
Cushing's syndrome
Pheochromocytoma
Acromegaly
Hyperparathyroidism
Neurological
Spinal cord disease
Raised intracranial pressure
Other
Coarction of the aorta
Pseudohypertension

Table 2.1

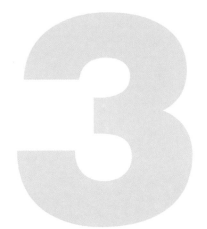

The need to treat: evidence from controlled clinical trials

Chapter 3

The need to treat: evidence from controlled clinical trials

Until 1985, hypertension in the elderly did not tend to be treated, mainly because it was feared that decreasing the blood pressure would increase episodes of orthostatic hypotension and/or induce coronary or cerebral thrombosis. These fears should have been dispelled 13 years before, when the U.S. Veterans Administration Cooperative Study Group on Antihypertensive Agents showed that stroke incidence fell by 70% in those over 60 years of age in whom hypertension was treated aggressively.[26] The findings of this trial were supported by various other studies (see below).

Australian Therapeutic Trial in Mild Hypertension

In the 1980 Australian Therapeutic Trial in Mild Hypertension, active treatment of patients (from 60 to 69 years of age) with hypertension produced 33% fewer strokes and 18% fewer coronary events than in the placebo group.[27]

European Working Party on High Blood Pressure in the Elderly

In 1985, the European Working Party on High Blood Pressure in the Elderly (EWPHE) results were published.[28] It followed 840 men and women (70% were women) over 60 years of age for a mean of 4.7 years and a maximum of 11 years *(Table 3.1)*. All had diastolic pressures of 90–119 mm Hg at entry and systolic pressures of 160–239 mm Hg. Treatment began with hydrochlorothiazide and triamterene, and methyldopa was added if the observed decrease in pressure was not

Table 3.1. EWPHE, European Working Party on High Blood Pressure in the Elderly; BP, blood pressure; SBP, systolic blood pressure; DBP, diastolic blood pressure.

EWPHE summary	
Number of patients	840 (70% women)
Age	> 60 years
Entry BP	SBP 160–239 mm Hg, DBP 90–119 mm Hg
Treatment	Hydrochlorothiazide/triamterene, adding methyldopa
Result	32% fewer stroke deaths, 38% fewer cardiac deaths

adequate. There were 32% fewer stroke deaths and 38% fewer cardiac deaths in the active treatment group than in the placebo group.

Coope and Warrender trial

In the 1986 Coope and Warrender trial, 884 patients of 60–79 years of age, with blood pressures of 160–230 mm Hg systolic or 105–120 mm Hg diastolic, were randomized to treatment with atenolol or placebo as first step treatment.[29] A second step of bendrofluazide or methyldopa was used if the first was not effective. The active treatment was associated with a reduction of 42% in stroke, of 15% in cardiac events, and of 23% in all cardiovascular events.

The Swedish Trial in Old Patients with Hypertension

The Swedish Trial in Old Patients with Hypertension trial (STOP-Hypertension) followed 1627 men and women who were 70–84 years of age for 1–4 years (mean of 25 months) *(Table 3.2)*.[30] They were required to have systolic pressures of 180–230 mm Hg with a diastolic pressures of over 90 mm Hg, or to have diastolic pressures of 105–120 mm Hg. Active treatment (in 812 patients) was with atenolol, metoprolol, pindolol, or hydrochlorothiazide, plus amiloride if necessary.

There were 40% fewer cardiovascular primary end points (p = 0.0031), 47% fewer fatal and non-fatal strokes (p = 0.0081), and a 42% reduction in total mortality (p = 0.0079) in the active treatment group, compared with placebo. There were 132 secondary end points (such as congestive heart failure, transient ischemic attacks, and angina) in the placebo group, compared with 40 in the active treatment group.

STOP-Hypertension found that lowering blood pressure was of benefit up to 80 years of age, with women benefiting as much as men. The results were so good that

STOP-Hypertension summary	
Number of patients	1627 men and women
Age	70–84 years
Entry BP	SBP 180–230 mm Hg, DBP 90–120 mm Hg
Treatment	Beta blockers or hydrochlorothiazide, adding amiloride
Result	40% fewer cardiovascular events, 47% fewer strokes, 42% lower mortality Benefit up to 84 years of age

Table 3.2 STOP-Hypertension, Swedish Trial in Old Patients with Hypertension; BP, blood pressure; SBP, systolic blood pressure; DBP, diastolic blood pressure.

the trial was stopped early by the safety committee. A later pharmaco-economic analysis of the results concluded that treating elderly men and women with diuretics and/or beta blockers is highly cost-effective.[31]

The subjects of these five initial trials were mainly patients with combined systolic and diastolic hypertension: when the trials were started, isolated systolic hypertension was not considered a risk. However, the following randomized, controlled trials included patients over 60 years of age with isolated systolic hypertension. All showed that antihypertensive treatment produced highly significant reductions in severe morbidity and in mortality.

The Medical Research Council Working Party Trial

The Medical Research Council (MRC) Working Party Trial was the first trial in the elderly to include patients with systolic hypertension.[32] It entered 4396 men and women who were 65–74 years of age into a comparison of amiloride, atenolol, and placebo (Table 3.3). Systolic blood pressure at entry had to be 160–209 mm Hg and diastolic pressure had to be < 115 mm Hg. Mean blood pressure at entry was 185/91 mm Hg. Both treatments reduced blood pressure to below the placebo level. Those on active treatment had 25% fewer strokes, 19% fewer coronary events, and a 17% drop in all cardiovascular events compared with placebo, but the benefit was only achieved by the diuretic. The difference between the diuretic and placebo in the number of adverse events was statistically significant (falls of 31% in stroke and 44% in coronary events on diuretic therapy): this was not so for the beta blocker (Table 3.4).

The Systolic Hypertension in the Elderly Programme

In the Systolic Hypertension in the Elderly Programme (SHEP), 4736 patients (57% women) of over 60 years of age (there was no upper age limit), with systolic pres-

MRC trial summary	
Number of patients	4396 men and women
Age	65–74 years
Entry BP	SBP 160–209 mm Hg, DBP< 115 mm Hg
Treatment	Amiloride, atenolol or placebo
Result	17% fewer cardiovascular events (but only with diuretic), 25% fewer strokes, 19% fewer coronary events

Table 3.3 MRC, Medical Research Council; BP, blood pressure; SBP, systolic blood pressure; DBP, diastolic blood pressure.

Events/1000 patient years in the MRC elderly trial			
	Group		
	Diuretic	**Atenolol**	**Placebo**
Total stroke	7.3	9.0	10.8
Total coronary	7.7	12.8**	12.7
All deaths	21.3	26.4*	24.7

Table 3.4 MRC, Medical Research Council. *p = 0.07. **p = 0.006, diuretic versus atenolol.

sures of 160–219 mm Hg and diastolic pressures < 90 mm Hg, were randomized to chlorthalidone 12.5 mg/day or placebo.[33] The dose was doubled if a satisfactory pressure was not achieved, and atenolol or reserpine were added if necessary.

The 5-year incidence of total stroke on active treatment was 5.2%, compared with 8.2% on placebo, a highly significant 36% reduction in risk (p = 0.0003). There were similar reductions in non-fatal myocardial infarction and coronary death (27%) and in major cardiovascular events (32%). The treatment allowed many older men and women to avoid intense cardiovascular interventions: the active treatment was associated with fewer coronary bypass grafts and percutaneous transluminal coronary angioplasties in patients under 75 years of age.

Systolic Hypertension in Europe Trial

The Systolic Hypertension in Europe trial (Syst-Eur[34]), like SHEP, concentrated on isolated systolic hypertension. It randomized 4695 patients (67% women), who were 70 years of age on average, to placebo or to nitrendipine as first-line treatment. If this failed to reduce the blood pressure satisfactorily, enalapril and hydrochlorothiazide were the second and third drugs of choice. The actively treated group had significantly fewer:

- Total strokes (by 42%).
- Non-fatal strokes (by 44%).
- All fatal and non-fatal cardiac end points (by 26%).
- All fatal and non-fatal cardiovascular events (by 31%).

During treatment, the blood pressures of the active and placebo treatment groups differed by 10.1/5 mm Hg (average blood pressure on placebo was 160.9/83.5 mm Hg and on active treatment was 150.8/78.5 mm Hg).

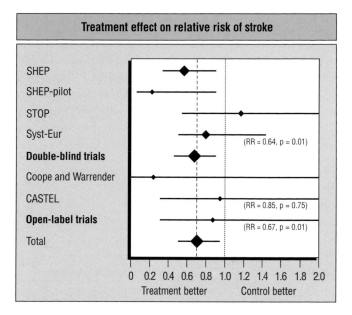

Figure 3.1 *Area of symbols is proportional to the amount of information provided. Error bars = 95% confidence interval. SHEP, Systolic Hypertension in the Elderly; STOP, Swedish Trial in Old Patients; Syst-Eur, Systolic hypertension in Europe; CASTEL, Cardiovascular study in the elderly; RR, relative risk.*

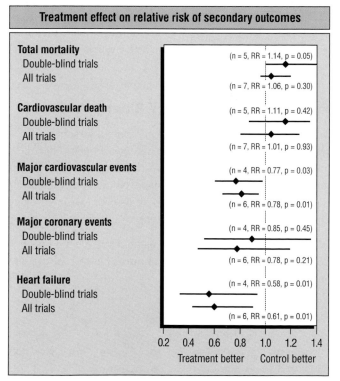

Figure 3.2 *Area of symbols is proportional to the amount of information provided. Error bars = 95% confidence interval. RR, relative risk; n, number of trials.*

Is there a cut-off age for starting treatment?

In March 1999, the Individual Data Analysis of Antihypertensive intervention (INDANA) group, representatives of the SHEP, STOP, EWPHE, Syst-Eur, and the Cardiovascular Study in the Elderly (CASTEL) trialists,[35] combined to collect data from all participants aged 80 years and over from their trials.[36] The effect of treatment on relative risk of stroke (the primary outcome) and of secondary outcomes (death from all causes, cardiovascular death, fatal and non-fatal major coronary and cardiovascular events, and heart failure) are shown in *Figures 3.1 and 3.2.*

The meta-analysis of data from 1670 participants 80 years of age or older suggested that treatment prevented 34% of strokes (95% CI 8–52). Major cardiovascular event rates were reduced by 22% and heart failure by 39%. However, there was no treatment benefit for cardiovascular death. There were 57 strokes and 34 deaths among 874 actively treated patients, compared with 77 strokes and 28 stroke deaths among 796 controls. This represents one non-fatal stroke prevented by treating about 100 very elderly patients with hypertension for a year.

The authors were struck by the contrast between the inconclusive findings for mortality and the benefit that treatment produced for non-fatal events. They concluded that a large-scale specific trial is needed before it can be proved that antihypertensive treatment is beneficial for the very old. However, they also stress that they cannot justify an age threshold beyond which hypertension cannot be treated.

Hypertension in the Very Elderly Trial

To date no single trial has recruited enough patients over 80 years of age to show a clear benefit from treatment. The number of people over 80 years of age is increasing and in many countries this group is the fastest growing group within the elderly. They are at a high risk of a cardiovascular event, with cardiovascular disease being the leading cause of death in Europe for both men and women. There is a need for a randomized controlled trial in this age group to assess the benefits of treatment and the risks.

With this in mind, the Hypertension in the Very Elderly Trial (HYVET) was started.[37] The pilot trial was stopped in June 1998 and the main trial will be starting in the summer of 1999.

The pilot study, which was of a PROBE (prospective, randomized, open-blinded end points) design, examined antihypertensive therapy in men and women over 80 years of age. It compared initial therapy with a diuretic or angiotensin-converting enzyme (ACE) inhibitor, with or without a calcium channel blocker, against no treatment in combined systolic and diastolic hypertension.

The main trial, which is of a double-blind design, is based on the success of the pilot and will compare treatment with the diuretic indapamide SR 1.5 mg against placebo. Clinical trials have confirmed a similar antihypertensive efficacy of indapamide SR in the short term and long term, both in monotherapy and in combination therapy, to other antihypertensive drugs, such as calcium channel blockers or ACE inhibitors.[38,39] The ACE inhibitor perindopril will be added as second-line therapy to achieve a target blood pressure of 150/80 mm Hg. The effects of these two agents are largely additive and the combination of an ACE inhibitor with a diuretic has been shown to be well tolerated in various patient groups. The trial plans to recruit 2100 patients and follow them up for an average of 5 years. It should help to establish the benefits and risks of treating the very elderly patient with hypertension.

Summary of all the trials

Tables 3.5 and 3.6 summarize the seven major trials of treatment of hypertension in the elderly.

The trials have established beyond doubt that combined systolic and diastolic hypertension must be treated at 60–80 years of age. Moreover, although the benefits of treating systolic hypertension are less in absolute terms, this must be treated in this age group. The authors are on record as stating:

> *'The trial data have shown that hypertension should be treated in all patients aged 65 to 80 years and BP values should be lowered below 160 and 90 mm Hg or probably lower for systolic and diastolic pressures, respectively. Lowering BP in the elderly has greater absolute benefits in terms of preventing stroke or coronary events compared with younger patients, as these are more frequent in the elderly.'* [40]

Does treatment of hypertension prevent dementia?

Preventing dementia in very elderly patients with hypertension

The main aim of treatment of hypertension has been to prevent or reduce the incidence of cardiovascular events, mainly stroke and myocardial infarction. However, one of the primary aims of the Syst-Eur trial (in which none of the patients initially had dementia) was to determine whether antihypertensive treatment reduces the incidence of dementia or alters cognitive function.[41] Significantly fewer cases of dementia occurred on active treatment with nitrendipine as first-line treatment than on placebo, but as the results were based on only 32 dementia events, the possible impact of the active treatment ranged from no effect to a 76% reduction in dementia rate and

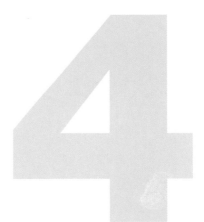

Making the diagnosis and initiating treatment

Chapter 4

Making the diagnosis and initiating treatment

The randomized, controlled clinical trials of drugs in hypertension in the elderly have established that lowering high blood pressure reduces the risk of cardiovascular events and death. However, there is more to treating hypertension than simply prescribing antihypertensive drugs. To begin with, the diagnosis of hypertension needs to be confirmed. This is not a matter of a single casual measurement, but of finding the pressure to be high on repeated measurement using a standard procedure, and recognising pitfalls such as white coat hypertension and the rare condition of pseudohypertension.

Once the diagnosis is made, a decision on whether to perform any further tests must be made before starting treatment. The treatment itself combines non-pharmaceutical advice and the use of antihypertensive agents, of which there is now an extensive choice.

Antihypertensive treatment according to concomitant diseases in elderly patients							
Coexisting pathology	Low dose diuretics	beta blockers	ACE inhib	AT2 antag	alpha blockers	Dihydro CCB	Benz CCB/ver
Asthma or COPD	++	CI	+	++	+	+	+
Heart failure	+	C	++	+	+	C	C/CI*
Angina	+	+	+	+	C	++	++
Past MI	+	++	++	+	C	C	C
Sick sinus syndrome	+	CI	+	+	+	+	CI
Peripheral vascular disease	+	C	+	+	++	++	++
Aortic stenosis	+	+	CI	C	+	CI	+
Renal failure + RAS	+	+	CI	C	+	+	+
Renal failure, no RAS	+	+	C	C	+	+	+
Prostatic hypertrophy	+	+	+	+	++	+	+
Diabetes mellitus	+	C	++	+	+	+	+
Dyslipidemia	+	C	+	+	+	+	+
Impotence	C	C	+	+	+	+	+
Gout	C	+	+	+	+	+	+
Constipation	+	+	+	+	+	+	+
Glaucoma	+	++	+	+	+	+	+

Table 4.1. Columns: ACE inhib., ACE inhibitors; AT2 antag., AT$_2$ receptor antagonists; Dihydro CCB, dihydropyridine calcium channel blockers; Benz CCB/ver, Benzothiazepine calcium channel blockers/verapamil. C/CI, Benz CCB=C, verapamil=CI. COPD, chronic obstructive pulmonary disease; MI, myocardial infarction; RAS, renal artery stenosis. ++, First-line drug; +, can be added; C, use with caution; CI, contraindicated.*

Elderly patients with hypertension often have other diseases and risk factors that may determine the type of drug that can or cannot be used *(Table 4.1)*. Side effects of such drugs may worsen the patient's quality of life: this is a major consideration in the elderly.

Making the diagnosis

Care must be taken, especially in the elderly, to take the blood pressure in a standard and reproducible way. If a mercury sphygmomanometer is used, the forearm should be supported and the antecubital fossa should be at the level of the heart. An appropriate cuff for the thickness of the arm should be used: it should be inflated to 30 mm Hg above the level at which the pulse disappears, then deflated slowly while the Korotkoff sounds are heard over the brachial artery. The systolic pressure is recorded as soon as the sound reappears, and the diastolic pressure is recorded at both the time of muffling of the sounds and the point at which they disappear. The pressure can be recorded to an accuracy of 2 mm Hg, and should not be rounded up or down to the nearest 5 mm Hg.

In white coat hypertension, the fact that the doctor is taking the reading causes the patient's blood pressure to be raised. It may be lower when the nurse takes it at home, but even then the effect may not be abolished.[51] If white coat hypertension is present, it is important to note that it may not be benign: patients with it are at higher risk for cardiovascular events than normotensive patients.[52] However, if a high pressure does become near-normal at home, unnecessary over-treatment can be avoided.

In pseudohypertension, the intra-arterial pressure is much lower than the cuff pressure reading because the brachial artery is heavily calcified, and therefore cannot be compressed. The artery below the cuff is still palpable when the cuff is inflated above the systolic pressure. Although it is very rare, pseudohypertension may lead to unnecessary treatment, and even to the misdiagnosis of malignant hypertension.[53] Patients whose blood pressure seems much higher than the clinical signs warrant should be considered candidates for it. X-ray confirmation of a calcified brachial artery and a much lower finger blood pressure measured by finger cuff occlusion will confirm the diagnosis.

Ambulatory blood pressure monitoring is only recommended for doubtful cases in whom white coat hypertension is suspected, or as a research tool. As yet, there are no prospective trials that link ambulatory blood pressure measurements (which are usually lower than office measurements) to prognosis.

Hypertension should be confirmed by at least three clinic measurements on different occasions a few weeks apart, unless the pressure is so high it is an emergency. The erect pressure and supine or sitting pressure should be recorded each time. In patients younger than 80 years of age, treatment should be started when the systolic pressure remains > 160 mm Hg.

Deciding on treatment

It is accepted that the higher the blood pressure, the higher the risk of stroke and ischemic heart disease.[54] However, lowering blood pressure is only one of many targets in most elderly patients, many of whom have complications from their lifetime of hypertension or have other diseases. For example, many have had previous cardiac events that require treatment with antithrombotics such as aspirin, or they have target-organ damage such as left ventricular hypertrophy or renal disease. Many smoke, are diabetic, have hyperlipidemias, are obese, and are extremely sedentary. Each of these factors adds to the risk of coronary and cerebrovascular events, and all need constant attention and proper management.

Elderly patients often find it difficult to comply with complicated treatment regimens, particularly if they involve multiple drugs and/or multiple doses. When the patient lives alone and may be mildly demented or depressed, compliance with such regimens becomes impossible. Treatment regimens must be kept simple, and as far as possible, factors that may raise blood pressure should be corrected non-pharmacologically before an antihypertensive drug is used.

Non-pharmacological treatment

This includes:

- Stopping smoking.
- Losing excess weight.
- Reducing alcohol intake.
- Eating less salt.

Although smoking raises blood pressure within minutes of lighting up,[55] it does not raise blood pressure in the long term. However, it does add to cardiovascular risk in people with hypertension,[33,56] so that it should be strongly discouraged and stopped if possible. The MRC trial in middle-aged patients showed that propranolol was less effective in lowering blood pressure and preventing cardiovascular events in smokers than in non-smokers.[32]

Weight reduction usually reduces blood pressure in obese patients,[57] sometimes to the extent that antihypertensive treatment is no longer necessary. This scenario is also observed in heavy drinkers who abstain.[58] Restricting salt intake is more successful in reducing blood pressure in the elderly than in younger patients,[59] and some people find this easier than stopping smoking or drinking alcohol.

Regular exercise can reduce blood pressure and maintain it at a lower level, but this option is not always open to or practical for many elderly people. However, in those that are capable, moderate exercise such as swimming and brisk walking can be of benefit and may improve the patient's quality of life.

Target blood pressures – forgetting the J-shaped curve

Over time, the targets for lowering blood pressures have changed and the long-standing argument about whether there is a 'J-shaped curve' for optimum blood pressure lowering has been resolved.

The J-shape controversy started when a 1987 study of 686 middle-aged men given a beta blocker or a thiazide diuretic demonstrated a blood pressure threshold of 150/90 mm Hg below which there was an increase in cardiac events.[60] The Coope and Warrender study[29] also found a J-shaped curve for diastolic pressure, while the EWPHE study did so for systolic pressure.[28] However, further analysis of the EWPHE subgroups showed that patients with the lowest systolic and diastolic pressures had more underlying illness than patients with higher pressures. In addition, the J-shaped curve was also observed in the placebo group. SHEP concluded that there was a J-shaped curve for systolic blood pressure and total mortality, but that reducing the diastolic pressure from 77 to 68 mm Hg lowered the incidence of myocardial infarction.[33]

It appears that the J-shaped curve is artificial, in that patients with the lowest systolic and diastolic pressures already have or develop more serious cardiovascular or other diseases than those with slightly higher blood pressures. In a relatively healthy person with mild to moderate hypertension, it appears that the lower the blood pressure, the better. However, excessive lowering of blood pressure in the elderly should be avoided, if only to prevent severe postural hypotension.

The current evidence suggests that the lower limits of target systolic and diastolic pressure should be 130 and 70 mm Hg in elderly patients, respectively *(Table 4.2)*. More realistic simple reading targets are 140/80–85 mm Hg. Ambulatory blood pressure readings can reduce these goals a little, as they tend to be lower than the corresponding clinic cuff measurement.

Target pressures in otherwise healthy elderly patients with hypertension		
	Blood pressures (mm Hg)	
Target	**Systolic**	**Diastolic**
Ideal	130	70
Realistic	140	80–85
NB Take sitting and standing blood pressures to prevent orthostatic hypotension. Ambulatory targets can be lower		

Table 4.2

Choosing an antihypertensive drug regimen for the elderly

Chapter 5

Choosing an antihypertensive drug regimen for the elderly

General principles

To ensure optimum compliance, antihypertensive therapy should be as simple as possible, especially in the elderly, who may have problems with concentration, understanding, and memory. The first-line therapy (as stated in the sixth report of the Joint National Committee on Prevention, Detection, Evaluation, and Treatment of High Blood Pressure [JNC VI]) should therefore be a single drug, preferably with a once-daily dosing regimen. In first-line treatment in uncomplicated hypertension a low dose diuretic or beta blocker should be used. In older patients with ISH, diuretics are preferred because they significantly reduced multiple end-point events; calcium antagonists could be appropriate alternatives in these patients. A second drug should only be tried as a substitute or an addition if the first choice drug is inadequate. Combinations of drugs do have advantages: they offer different but complementary ways of lowering pressure while minimizing side effects as they can be given in low doses.

Combining a diuretic with an ACE inhibitor, a beta blocker, an alpha blocker, or a calcium channel blocker is additive in lowering blood pressure.[61] Other proven additive combinations include a beta blocker plus an alpha blocker or plus a dihydropyridine calcium channel blocker, and an ACE inhibitor plus a calcium channel blocker.[61]

Starting patients on antihypertensive treatment involves frequent follow-up checks in subsequent weeks until the blood pressure is controlled. During this time, patients often need psychological support as they begin to realize that they will be on treatment, and will need regular checks, for the rest of their lives. When blood pressure is stable, the follow-up intervals can be lengthened to 3–4 months.

Patients on some regimens require regular laboratory tests. In those taking diuretics and/or ACE inhibitors, renal function monitoring is required for the first few months and then yearly thereafter. Once treatment is started, most patients will remain on it for life. However, a few (such as those who have changed their lifestyles for the better) may eventually be weaned off it.

The drugs

Diuretics

Diuretics remain the mainstay of antihypertensive treatment in the elderly. They reduce blood pressure first by reducing extracellular fluid volume, then by vasodilatation, and finally by reduction of intravascular fluid volume.[62] Their blood pressure lowering effects are well established, and their ability to prevent cardiovascular events proven, as they were used in all of the main randomized, controlled trials of antihypertensive agents in the elderly. They are cheap, well tolerated, and highly effective. The longer-acting diuretics are preferred in hypertension.

Commonly used thiazides include bendrofluazide, which can be used either alone, or in conjunction with a potassium sparing diuretic. The thiazide-related indapamide SR 1.5 mg has been shown to induce a reduction in left ventricular hypertrophy; this regression is obtained as a result of a reduction of wall thickness[63], and it produces no significant disturbance of lipid and glucose metabolism[64]. Indapamide SR 1.5 mg is a once-daily preparation with 24-hour activity.[65]

Diuretics trial results in the elderly

Diuretics and, to a lesser extent, beta blockers and calcium channel blockers are the only classes of drugs that have been shown to reduce overall cardiovascular morbidity and mortality. Indeed, a large body of evidence on the benefit of antihypertensive treatment in the elderly comes from diuretics. They were used as first-line treatment in the Australian Trial in Mild Hypertension, EWPHE, STOP-H, MRC, and SHEP, and as add-on treatment in the Coope and Warrender trial, STOP-H, and MRC.

The use of diuretics to lower blood pressures and cardiovascular events was reported in the EWPHE, SHEP, and MRC trials. The last of these concluded that hydrochlorothiazide and amiloride, but not atenolol, significantly reduced myocardial infarction in elderly patients with hypertension.

Side effects

Metabolic disturbances may occur with high-dose diuretic drug use. Low-dose thiazide diuretic drugs incur these problems to a lesser extent and so the frequency of adverse events is not as great. Hypokalemia, hypomagnesemia, disturbance of serum lipids [66], glucose [67] and uric acid [68] are much less commonly encountered than with high-dose diuretic medications. Indeed, major outcome trials have shown there is no relationship between low-dose thiazide use and sudden death due to arrythmias; notably, in the MRC trial the reduction in cardiac events was found in the diuretic treatment group, not in the beta-blocker treatment group. Hypokalemia is a concern when prescribing thiazide diuretics, for some patients, and a potassium supplement may be warranted. For patients taking digoxin or other QT-interval prolonging drugs, a potassium-sparing diuretic may be preferable. Acute gout is a potential side effect of thiazide diuretic drug use; the MRC and EWPHE trials have shown values of one instance per 250 patient years for this condition for patients receiving these drugs.

Low-dose thiazide diuretics offer great benefits in terms of cardiac risk reduction and whilst minor elevations of blood glucose and uric acid are sometimes seen with these drugs, these metabolic modulations have not been seen to be harmful, especially compared with the benefits reaped from their cardioprotective action. As elderly patients may be less able to eliminate drugs from their bodies renally, blood concentrations of diuretic drugs may be elevated for longer periods and low-dosage diuretics are indicated for these patients, as shown in *Table 5.1*.

Commonly recommended doses of diuretic drugs in elderly patients with hypertension	
Drug	**Dose (mg/day)**
Bendrofluazide	1.25–2.5
Chlorothiazide	500–1000
Chlorthalidone	25–50
Hydrochlorothiazide	12.5–25
Indapamide SR	1.5

Table 5.1

Beta blockers

Beta blockers lower blood pressure by reducing cardiac output, readjusting baroreceptor responses, decreasing renin release from the renal cortex, and reducing peripheral resistance: some may also have a central antihypertensive effect.[69]

All beta blockers are effective antihypertensive agents, but they vary widely with regard to their:

- Selectivity for beta-1 and beta-2 adrenoceptors.
- Intrinsic sympathomimetic activity (ISA).
- Membrane-stabilizing activity.
- Lipid solubility.
- Pharmacokinetics, including their lipid or water solubility and their duration of action.

Short-acting drugs are now presented in slow release preparations so that, like the longer acting drugs, they can be given once daily, which is essential for good compliance in the elderly.

First generation beta blockers (such as propranolol and oxprenolol) are not cardioselective. They produce symptomatic side effects and may produce peripheral ischemia and bronchoconstriction and reduce exercise tolerance. In addition to this, they may adversely affect lipid and glucose metabolism. As with all beta blockers, they are contraindicated in patients with asthma and should be used with caution in patients with type 1 diabetes.

Second generation beta blockers (such as atenolol, bisoprolol, and metoprolol) are more cardioselective, but they still have an adverse effect on lipid profiles. The third generation drugs, including celiprolol, are peripheral vasodilators and have no effect on lipid profiles.

Beta blockers with ISA (such as acebutolol, oxprenolol, and pindolol) are less likely to cause cold extremities (often an important feature in the elderly), and have less effect on cardiac output and resting heart rate. Those beta blockers that possess low lipid solubility, such as atenolol, are relatively free of central nervous system side effects. Combined alpha and beta receptor antagonists (such as carvedilol and labetalol) do not constrict the peripheral vessels, and have no effect on lipid levels.

Beta blocker trial results in the elderly

The Coope and Warrender trial concluded that atenolol prevents strokes but not heart disease in the elderly.[29] This was confirmed by the MRC trial result, in which atenolol did not lower myocardial infarction rates in elderly patients with hypertension.[32] When, in the SHEP study, low-dose chlorthalidone was used as first-line treatment and atenolol or reserpine were used as second-line treatment, strokes and coronary events were prevented.[33] Why beta blockers on their own may not prevent coronary events is not fully understood. It may be related to their effects on lipids and glucose metabolism, but this is still unproven.

Side effects of beta blockers in the elderly

Side effects of beta blockers in the elderly include bronchospasm (in patients with chronic obstructive lung disease and asthma) and Raynaud's phenomenon. Celiprolol may be an exception but more trials are needed to confirm this.

Older people with impaired left ventricular function may develop heart failure while taking beta blockers. Other side effects include central nervous symptoms such as dreams, hallucinations, and insomnia: the exceptions here are the water-soluble drugs such as atenolol and sotalol. Patients with mild cognitive effects may develop memory defects[70] and confusion[71] on propranolol, which, along with other beta blockers, can also cause mild depression in older patients with hypertension.[72]

Among the lipid changes associated with beta blockers in the elderly, are a rise of 20–30% in plasma triglycerides and a fall in high-density lipoprotein (HDL) cholesterol. As beta blockers are protective in heart disease, it is difficult to understand how these changes can be clinically relevant in the elderly.[73] The same reservation holds for the impaired glucose tolerance with which the non-cardioselective beta blockers are linked. Beta blockers reduce renal flow and glomerular filtration[74], and as such can further impair renal function in older people with established renal disease.

Other side effects of beta blockers include gastrointestinal upset, weight gain, and impotence. However, the side effects most likely to affect most patients' quality of life are fatigue, poor exercise tolerance, and cold extremities.

The recommended doses of beta blockers for the elderly person with hypertension are given in *Table 5.2*. It is best to start with at a low dose and increase gradually. If the treatment is to be stopped, this should also be done by decreasing the dose gradually.

Commonly recommended doses of beta blockers in elderly patients with hypertension	
Drug	**Dose**
Acebutolol	400 mg od or bid
Atenolol	50 mg od
Bisoprolol	10–20 mg od
Celiprolol	200–400 mg od
Metoprolol	100–200 mg od
Oxprenolol	80–240 mg bid
Pindolol	15–45 mg od

Table 5.2 od, once daily; bid, twice daily.

Angiotensin-converting enzyme inhibitors

ACE inhibitors lower blood pressure by blocking the conversion of inactive angiotensin I to the active vasoconstrictor angiotensin II. They are particularly effective in patients with congestive heart failure. Their effect is enhanced by sodium restriction or co-prescription with diuretics. They do not affect lipid or glucose metabolism.

They are all effective antihypertensive agents, but, like drugs in other categories, differ in their pharmacokinetics. Most are excreted renally but others may be excreted by the liver (eg, fosinopril).

Long-acting ACE inhibitors include fosinopril, lisinopril, perindopril, quinapril, and ramipril.

So far, there are no long-term controlled trial data on mortality and morbidity for ACE inhibitors as first-line treatment in elderly patients with hypertension.

Side effects of ACE inhibitors

When the first ACE inhibitor (captopril) was introduced, it was given in what are now known to be unnecessarily high doses. This led to many reports of rashes, loss of taste, and (less often) neutropenia; the latter occurring mainly in patients with renal disease or in those who were also receiving post-transplant or immunosuppressant therapy.

At today's lower doses, the most troublesome side effect is a dry cough. A more serious, but rarer side effect is the induction of renal failure in patients with renal artery stenosis of their one functioning kidney or of both kidneys. Kidney function is dependent on a high angiotensin II level, production of which is blocked by the drug treatment. Before considering an ACE inhibitor, renal artery bruit should be listened for in all patients, as the elderly are more likely than younger patients to have renal artery stenosis from atherosclerosis. They are also more likely than their younger counterparts to be dehydrated, to be taking diuretics, or to be in heart failure – all of which could result in severe hypotension if an ACE inhibitor is added.

Commonly recommended doses of ACE inhibitors in elderly patients with hypertension	
Drug	**Dose**
Captopril	6.25–50 mg tds
Enalapril	2.5–40 mg od
Fosinopril	10–40 mg od
Lisinopril	2.5–40 mg od
Perindopril	2–8 mg od
Quinapril	2.5–40 mg od
Ramipril	1.25–10 mg od

Table 5.3 ACE, angiotensin-converting enzyme; od, once daily; tds, three times per day.

Therefore, it is best to check renal function in an elderly patient before starting an ACE inhibitor. In patients with heart failure, a low dose of a short-acting ACE inhibitor should be tried first under medical supervision in hospital, where severe hypotension can be managed in an emergency.

The usual doses of the common ACE inhibitors are listed in *Table 5.3*.

Angiotensin-II antagonists

The angiotensin-II (AT-II) antagonists (candesartan, irbesartan, losartan, and valsartan) have a similar, but not identical action to ACE inhibitors. They directly antagonize angiotensin II at its receptor site and have less effect on bradykinin levels. As such, they do not produce the dry cough at therapeutic doses that accompanies the use of ACE inhibitors. As with ACE inhibitors, there are no published large long-term controlled trials of AT-II antagonists in hypertension. It has been suggested that these drugs should be limited to those with respiratory problems and to those who develop a cough on an ACE inhibitor.

Calcium channel blockers

Intracellular calcium is essential to smooth muscle contraction. By preventing calcium entry into vascular smooth muscle cells, calcium channel blockers reduce vascular tone, lowering peripheral resistance and blood pressure accordingly. The calcium channel blockers in current use act upon two main types of channel, classified as potential-mediated (L-type) or receptor-mediated. They have been divided pharmacologically into three groups:

- Verapamil, which stands on its own in blocking receptor-mediated channels. It is used more for heart arrhythmias than for hypertension, largely because its depressant action on cardiac function can precipitate heart failure if there is unsuspected disease of the conducting system or if it is co-prescribed with beta blockers. It also produces constipation in many subjects.

- Dihydropyridines (DHPs), such as amlodipine, felodipine, isradipine, lacidipine, lercanidipine, nicardipine, nifedipine, nisoldipine, and nitrendipine, have a more peripheral site of action than verapamil and are more appropriate anti-hypertensive agents. Early doubts about the safety of dihydropyridines (they were reported to cause a significant excess of deaths from myocardial infarction in patients with angina or recent myocardial infarction) have been dispelled.[75] These adverse reactions were linked with short-acting DHPs, dose regimens of which allowed periods of 'rebound' sympathetic activity with tachycardia. Now that long-acting, once daily preparations with 24-hour activity (amlodipine, felodipine, sustained release nifedipine) are available, this is no longer a concern.

- Benzothiazepines (including diltiazem) are the third group of calcium channel blockers. More like verapamil than the DHPs in its effect on the heart, diltiazem is primarily an antianginal drug, but also has a useful antihypertensive effect. Co-prescription of diltiazem with digoxin raises serum digoxin levels.

Trials of calcium channel blockers in the elderly

Two major trials have shown that DHP calcium channel blockers are effective in the elderly.

In the Shanghai Trial of Nifedipine in the Elderly (STONE), 1632 patients who were 60–79 years of age, with systolic or diastolic hypertension, were given nifedipine 10–60 mg or placebo twice daily.[76] There was a significant reduction in strokes and severe arrhythmias in the nifedipine group and this drug was recommended for elderly patients with hypertension.

Syst-Eur found that nitrendipine reduced the incidence of stroke by 42% and reduced cardiac events by 26% in 4695 elderly men and women with systolic hypertension.[32]

Side effects of calcium channel blockers

The most common problem with verapamil is constipation. Other reported side effects, such as fatigue, vomiting, bradycardia and heart block, gingival hyperplasia, gynecomastia, and reversible liver function test abnormalities, are rare. It is contraindicated in patients with bradycardia.

DHPs tend to cause flushing and tachycardia, but these are less common with the long-acting preparations. Ankle edema that does not respond to diuretics may be a problem in up to 10% of patients, but their peripheral vasodilatation is advantageous in patients with Raynaud's phenomenon. Diltiazem, like verapamil, causes brady-cardia, and is contraindicated in patients with bradycardia, left ventricular failure, heart block, or sick sinus syndrome. It can cause malaise, headache, flushes, gas-trointestinal upsets, altered liver function tests, and depression.

Commonly recommended doses of calcium channel blockers in elderly patients with hypertension	
Drug	**Dose**
Amlodipine	5–10 mg od
Diltiazem	200 mg od
Felodipine	5–20 mg od
Nicardipine	30 mg bid
Nifedipine	30–60 mg od
Verapamil	120–240 mg bid

Table 5.4 *od, once daily; bid, twice daily.*

Sudden cessation of therapy with calcium channel blockers may precipitate angina in susceptible patients. If they are to be withdrawn, this should be done gradually.

With increasing age, the elimination half-lives of verapamil and diltiazem lengthen, so the dose should be reduced accordingly. This is not necessary with the long-acting DHPs. *Table 5.4* gives the recommended doses of calcium antagonists in the elderly.

Alpha-1 blockers

Alpha blockers lower blood pressure by blocking the postsynaptic alpha receptors on vascular smooth muscle cells, thereby dilating peripheral arteries and veins, and decreasing peripheral resistance. Both terazosin and doxazosin have been shown to reduce symptoms of benign prostate hypertrophy.

Alpha blockers also affect blood lipid profiles in a positive way: in a meta-analysis of the treatment of 5413 patients with hypertension, monotherapy with doxazosin (in a cohort of 3000 patients) reduced low-density lipoprotein (LDL) cholesterol by 4.8%, reduced triglycerides by 7.6%, and increased the HDL:total cholesterol ratio by 5.8%.[77]

Side effects of alpha blockers

Prazosin, the first alpha blocker, was initially difficult to use because of its dramatic first dose effect. Blood pressures dropped precipitously after one dose, probably due to a huge reduction in venous return from the vasodilated periphery. One in five patients in these early trials developed orthostatic hypotension.[78] To avoid such reactions, alpha blockers must be started at their minimum dose, and titrated upwards slowly, at the same time withdrawing any previously prescribed diuretics.

Adverse effects of alpha blockers include headache, drowsiness, lethargy, weakness, impotence, palpitations, and nausea. Doxazosin has been linked with diarrhea, dyspnea, rhinitis, and non-anginal chest pain in a small number of patients.

The recommended doses of the current alpha blockers are given in *Table 5.5*.

Common drug interactions between antihypertensive agents and other drugs commonly used by the elderly

It is relatively simple to treat hypertension in an elderly patient if it is his or her only problem, and the first choice of drug will usually be a diuretic. However, many older patients are taking other drugs for common concomitant diseases, such as heart failure, ischemic heart disease, chronic lung disease, peripheral vascular disease, prostatic hypertrophy, diabetes, gout, impotence, constipation, and glaucoma. The choice of antihypertensive drug often depends on whether it may make one of these conditions worse. *Table 5.6* lists common harmful drug interactions in elderly patients given antihypertensive drugs.

Table 5.5 od, once daily; bid, twice daily.

Commonly recommended doses of alpha blockers in elderly patients with hypertension	
Drug	**Dose**
Doxazosin	1–16 mg od
Prazosin	0.5 mg daily to 10 mg bid

The most frequent potentially-hazardous drug interactions with antihypertensive drugs in the elderly								
	Digoxin	Amiodarone	Oral anti-diabetics	NSAIDs	Dopa-minergics (levadopa)	Alpha blockers	Beta blockers	Diuretics K+ sparing
K+-losing diuretics	↑A (if ↓K+)	↑A (if ↓K+)	–	↑DRF	↑OH	↑OH	–	
ACE inhibitors	–	–	↑HE	↑DRF/AHE	↑OH	↑OH	–	↑K+
Beta blockers	↑AVB	↑AVB	↑HE	AHE	–	–	–	–
Alpha blockers	–		–	AHE	–		–	–
Calcium channel blockers								
Dihydropyridine	↑PC	–	–	AHE	↑OH	↑OH	–	–
Verapamil	↑AVB	↑AVB	–	AHE	–	–	↑AVB	–
Benzothiazepines	↑PC	↑AVB	–	AHE	–	–	↑AVB	–

Table 5.6 NSAID, non-steroidal anti-inflammatory drug; ↑, increased risk of or increased level of; A, arrhythmias; DRF, deterioration of renal function; OH, orthostatic hypotension (mainly when starting drugs); ACE, angiotensin-converting enzyme; HE, hypoglycemic effect; AHE, anagonize hypotensive effect; K+, potassium; AVB, atrio-ventricular block; PC, plasma concentration.

Tailoring the treatment –
a summary

Chapter 6

Tailoring the treatment – a summary

When an elderly patient has uncomplicated essential hypertension, the choice of treatment is easy; it should in the first place be a low-dose diuretic. Indeed, the World Health Organization–International Society of Hypertension (WHO–ISH) guidelines state that a compelling indication for the use of diuretics is advanced age.[79] They go on to state that they are 'inexpensive, effective, generally well tolerated in low doses' and 'have been clearly shown to prevent major cardiovascular events in a variety of patient groups'. The JNC-VI guidelines reiterate that if there are no specific indications for another type of drug 'in the elderly, diuretics should be chosen'.[80] If this does not lower the blood pressure adequately, then a beta blocker, ACE inhibitor, calcium channel blocker, or angiotensin II inhibitor may be added, as necessary.

This choice of therapy is less clear cut in patients with concomitant diseases, such as heart failure, ischemic heart disease, chronic lung disease, peripheral vascular disease, prostatic hypertrophy, diabetes, gout, constipation, glaucoma, and impotence, all of which may be affected, positively or negatively by the various drugs (Chapter 5).

The hemodynamic changes that occur with age, too, may affect the decision on how to treat. A lower stroke volume and an impaired baroreceptor reflex may make the elderly more susceptible than younger people to postural hypotension. Whatever drug is to be used, it is best to start with the lowest dose to avoid postural hypotension and other adverse effects.

Is there a cut-off age beyond which patients should not be treated? This question may not be answered until the results of the HYVET study are known. In their meta-analysis, the INDANA group concluded that, although an age threshold beyond which hypertension should not be treated cannot be justified, a large-scale specific study is needed for a definite conclusion to be drawn on whether antihypertensive treatment is beneficial in very elderly patients with hypertension. However, this does not mean that treatment should be stopped when people who have responded satisfactorily to antihypertensive therapy reach their 80th birthday. There is unlikely to be any harm, and there is probably benefit, in them continuing with their treatment.

In the meantime, all patients 60–80 years of age with established hypertension should be offered the benefits of treatment.

Conclusion

Lowering blood pressure in the elderly has greater absolute benefits in terms of preventing stroke or coronary events compared with younger patients, as they are more frequent in the elderly. Diuretics are still the first choice drug in uncomplicated hypertension and the least expensive. Other drug classes may be employed in the presence of concomitant diseases and/or drug treatments.[40]

References

1. O'Brien AAJ, Bulpitt CJ. In *The Encylopedia of Aging*. New York: Springer Publishing Company, 1995.

2. Kaplan N. **Primary hypertension.** In *Pathogenesis in Clinical Hypertension, 7th ed.* Williams and Wilkins, 1998;41–100.

3. Starr JM, Bulpitt CJ. **Hypertension.** In *Epidemiology of Old Age*. Edited by S Ebrahim. London: BMJ Publishing Group, 1996.

4. Kannel WB. **Hypertension and the risk of cardiovascular disease.** In *Hypertension: Pathophysiology, Diagnosis, and Management.* Edited by Laragh JH, Brenner BM. New York: Raven Press, 1990, 101–117.

5. Tsang KWT, Bulpitt CJ. **Hypertension.** In *Drug Therapy in Old Age*. Edited by CF George, MJ Woodhouse MJ, *et al.* John Wiley & Sons Ltd; 1999.

6. Drizd T, Dannenberg AL, Engel A. **Blood pressure levels in persons 18–74 years of age in 1976–80, and trends in blood pressure from 1960 to 1980 in the United States.** In *Vital Health Statistics Series, Hyattsville, Maryland: U.S.* Department of Health and Human Services: DHHS publication no (PHS), 1986; 11:86–1684.

7. Hypertension Detection Follow-Up Cooperation Group. **Five year findings of the Hypertension Detection Follow-up Program.** *JAMA* 1979, **242**:2562–2571.

8. OPCS Social Survey Division. *Health Survey for England 1993*. London: HMSO; 1994.

9. Royal College of General Practitioners, Office of Population Censuses and Surveys, Department of Health and Social Security. *Morbidity Statistics from General Practice 1981-82, series MB5 No 1*. London: HMSO; 1986.

10. Bulpitt CJ. **Definition, prevalence and incidence of hypertension in the elderly.** In *Handbook of Hypertension, Hypertension in the Elderly*, 1989; 12:155–169.

11. Shaper AG, Wright DM, Kyobe J. **Blood pressure and body build in three nomadic tribes of northern Kenya.** *East Afr Med J* 1969, **46**:273–281.

12. Elliott P. **Observational studies on salt and blood pressure.** *Hypertension* 1991, **7**:13–18.

13. Law MR, Frost CD, Wald NJ. **By how much does dietary salt reduction lower blood pressure? I and II: Analysis of observational data within populations.** *Br Med J* 1991, **312**:811–818.

14. Dyer AR, Elliott P. **The INTERSALT study: relations of body mass index to blood pressure.** *J Hum Hypertens* 1989, **3**:299–308.

15. Fagard RH. **Physical fitness and blood pressure.** *J Hypertens* 1993, **11** (suppl 5):547–552.

16. Paffenberger RS, Wing AL, Hyde RT, *et al.* **Physical activity and incidence of hypertension in college alumni.** *Am J Epidemiol* 1983, **117**:245–257.

17. World Hypertension League. **Alcohol and hypertension: implications for management.** *Bull World Health Organ* 1991, **69**:377–382.

18. Klatsky AL, Friedman GD, Spieglaub AB, *et al.* **Alcohol consumption and blood pressure. Kaiser Permanente Multiphasic Health Examination Data.** *N Engl J Med* 1977, **296**:1194–2000.

19. Fortmann SP, Haskell WL, Vranizan K, *et al.* **The association of blood pressure and dietary alcohol: differences by age, sex and oestrogen use.** *Am J Epidemiol* 1983, **118**:497–507.

20. Staessen J, Amery A, Fagard R. **Isolated systolic hypertension in the elderly.** *J Hypertens* 1990, **8**:393–405.

21. Tarazi RC, Martini F, Dustan HP. **The role of aortic distensibility in hypertension.** In *International Symposium on Hypertension.* Edited by P Milliez, M Sasar. Monaco: Boehringer Ingelheim; 1975.

22. Zemel MB, Sower JR. **Salt sensitivity and systolic hypertension in the elderly.** *Am J Cardiol* 1988, **61**:7H–12H.

23. Abrass IB. **Catecholamine levels and vascular responsiveness in ageing.** In *Relation and Ageing, an NIH Symposium.* Biomedical Information Corporation: New York; 1986.

24. Fleich JH, Malin HM, Brodie BB. **Beta-receptor activity in an artery. Variation in age and species.** *Circ Res* 1970, **26**:151–162.

25. Furchgott RF, Zawadki JV. **The obligatory role of endothelial cells in relaxation of arterial smooth muscle by acetylcholine.** *Nature* 1980, **299**:373–376.

26. Veterans Administration Cooperative Study Group on Antihypertensive Agents. Report 1972.

27. Australian Therapeutic Trial Management Committee. **The Australian therapeutic trial in mild hypertension.** *Lancet* 1980, **i**:1261–1267.

28. Amery A, Birkenhager WH, Bulpitt CJ, *et al.* **The European Working Party on High blood pressure in the Elderly. Proceedings of a symposium held in Rome, 19–20 November 1989.** *Am J Med* 1991, **90** (suppl 3A):1S–64S.

29. Coope J, Warrender TS. **Randomised trial of treatment of hypertension in elderly patients in primary care.** *Br Med J* 1986, **293**:1145–1151.

30. Dahlof B, Hansson L, Lindholm LH, *et al.* **Swedish trial in old patients with hypertension (STOP-Hypertension): analysis performed up to 1992.** *Clin Exp Hypertens* 1993, **15**:925–939.

31. Johanesson M, Dahlof B, Lindholm LH, *et al.* **The cost-effectiveness of treating hypertension in elderly people – an analysis of the Swedish Trial in Old Patients with Hypertension (STOP-Hypertension).** *J Intern Med* 1993, **234**:317–323.

32. The MRC Working Party. **Medical Research Council trial of treatment of hypertension in older adults: principal results.** *Br Med J* 1992, **304**:405–412.

33. SHEP Cooperative Research Group. **Prevention of stroke by antihypertensive drug treatment in older persons with isolated systolic hypertension. Final results of the Systolic Hypertension in the Elderly Program (SHEP).** *JAMA* 1991, **265**:3255–3264.

34. Staessen J, Fagard R, Thijs L, *et al.* **Randomised double-blind comparison of placebo and active treatment for older patients with isolated systolic hypertension.** *Lancet* 1997, **350**:757–764.

35. Casiglia E, Spolaore P, Mazza A, *et al.* **Effect of two different therapeutic approaches on total and cardiovascular mortality in a cardiovascular study in the elderly (CASTEL).** *Jpn Heart J* 1994, **35**:589–600.

36. Gueyffier F, Bulpitt C, Boissel J-P, *et al.* **Antihypertensive drugs in very old people: a subgroup meta-analysis of randomised controlled trials.** *Lancet* 1999, **353**:793–796.

37. Bulpitt CJ, Fletcher AE, Amery A, *et al.* **The Hypertension in the Very Elderly Trial (HYVET). Rationale, methodology and comparison with previous trials.** *Drugs Aging* 1994, **5**:171–183.

38. Guez D, Mallion JM, Degaute JP, *et al.* **Low dose antihypertensive therapy with indapamide 1.5mg sustained release coated tablets: pooled data from two European multicenter randomized double blind studies in 690 patients.** *Arch Mal Coeur Vaiss* 1996, **89**:17–26.

39. Bulpitt CJ, Emeriau JP, Knauf H, *et al.* **Equivalence study of antihypertensive effect of indapamide sustained-release (SR) 1.5 mg, Hydrochlorothiazide 25 mg and amlodipine 5 mg in hypertension.** *J Hypertens* 1997, **15**(suppl 14):S130.

40. Bonapace S, Rajkumar C, Bulpitt CJ. **Tailoring anti-hypertensive treatment in the elderly.** *J Hum Hypertens* 1998, **12**:615–620.

41. Forette F, Seux ML, Staessen JA, *et al.* **Prevention of dementia in randomised double blind placebo controlled Systolic Hypertension in Europe (Syst-Eur) trial.** *Lancet* 1998, **352**:1347–1351.

42. Pahor M, Somes GW, Franse LV *et al.* **Prevention of dementia: Syst-Eur trial (letter).** *Lancet* 1999, **353**:253

43. Zuccalà G, Pedone C, Cocchi A, *et al.* **Prevention of dementia: Syst-Eur trial (letter).** *Lancet* 1999, **353**:253–254.

44. Skook I, Lernfelt B, Landahl S, *et al.* **15-years longitudinal study of blood pressure and dementia.** *Lancet* 1996, **347**:1141–1145.

45. Pasquier F, Leys D. **Why are stroke patients prone to develop dementia?** *J Neurol* 1997, **244**:135–142.

46. Kario K, Pickering TG. **Calcium antagonists and prevention of dementia in elderly people.** *Lancet* 1999, **353**:1184.

47. Sevush S, Jy W, Horstmann LL, *et al.* **Platelet activation in Alzheimer's disease.** *Arch Neurol* 1998, **55**:530–536.

48. Skoog I. **The relationship between blood pressure and dementia: a review.** *Biomed Pharmacother* 1997, **51**:367–375.

49. Shirohase H, Suzuki Y, Kunitomo K *et al.* ***In vitro* inhibition of platelet aggregation by indapamide (Natrilix).** *J Med Pharm Sci* 1987, **18**:1021–1024.

50. Lebel M, Gbeassor FM, Grose JH. **Role of prostanoids in the antihypertensive action of indapamide.** *Drugs Today* 1989, **25**(suppl. 11):53–58.

51. Mancia G, Parati G, Pomidossi G, *et al.* **Alerting reaction and rise in blood pressure during measurement by physician and nurse.** *Hypertension* 1987, **9**:209–215.

52. Julius S, Jamerson K, Gudbrandsson T, *et al.* **White coat hypertension: a follow up.** *Clin Exp Hypertens [A]* 1992, **14**:45–53.

53. Littenberg B, Wolfberg C. **Pseudohypertension masquerading as malignant hypertension. Case report and review of the literature.** *Am J Med* 1988, **84**:539–542

54. MacMahon S, Peto R, Cutler J, *et al.* **Blood pressure, stroke and coronary heart disease. Part 1: Prolonged differences in blood pressure: prospective observational studies corrected for the regression dilution bias.** *Lancet* 1990, **335**:765–774.

55. Baer L, Radichevich I. **Cigarette smoking in hypertensive patients. Blood pressure and endocrine responses.** *Am J Med* 1985, **78**:564–568.

56. Bulpitt CJ, Beilin LJ, Clifton P, *et al.* **Risk factors for death in treated hypertensive patients.** *Lancet* 1979, **2**:134–137.

57. MacMahon SW, MacDonald GJ, Berstein L, *et al.* **Comparison of weight reduction with metoprolol in treatment of hypertension in young overweight patients.** *Lancet* 1985, **1**:1233–1236.

58. Potter JF, Beevers DG. **Pressor effect of alcohol in hypertension.** *Lancet* 1984, **1**:119–122.

59. Myers J, Morgan T. **The effects of sodium intake on the blood pressure related to age and sex.** *Clin Exp Hypertens* 1983, **A5**:99–118.

60. Cruikshank JM, Thorp JM, Zacharias FJ. **Benefits and potential harm of lowering blood pressure.** *Lancet* 1987, **1**:581–584.

61. Letzel H, Bluemner E. **Dose–response curves in antihypertensive combination therapy: results of a controlled clinical trial.** *J Hypertens* 1990, **8** (suppl 4):S83–S86.

62. Shah S, Khatri I, Feis ED. **Mechanism of antihypertensive effect of thiazide diuretics.** *Am Heart J* 1978, **95**:611–618.

63.Gosse P, Dubourg O, Gueret P, *et al.* **Regression of left ventricular hypertrophy in hypertensive patients treated with indapamide SR 1.5 versus enalapril: results of L.I.V.E. study.** *J Am Coll Cardiol* 1999, **33**(suppl. A): 246.

64. Ambrosioni E, Safar M, Degaute JP, *et al.* **Low-dose antihypertensive therapy with 1.5mg sustained-release indapamide: results of randomised double-blind controlled studies.** *J Hypertens* 1998, **16**:1677–1684

65. Mallion JM, Asmar R, Boutelant S, *et al.* **Twenty-four hour antihypertensive efficacy of indapamide, 1.5-mg sustained relcase: results of two randomized double-blind controlled studies.** *J Cardiovasc Pharmacol* 1998, **32**: 673–678.

66. Ames RP. **The effects of anti-hypertensive drugs on serum lipids and lipoproteins. Part 1. Diuretics.** *Drugs* 1986, **32**:260–278.

67. Moser M. **Updates on some hypertensive treatment controversies.** *Cardiovasc Risk Factors* 1991, **1**:413–426.

68. Langford HG, Blaufox D, Borhani NO, *et al.* **Is thiazide-produced uric acid elevation harmful? Analysis of data from the Hypertension Detection and Follow up program.** *Arch Intern Med* 1987, **147**:645–649.

69. Prichard BNC. **Propranolol and beta-adrenergic receptor blocking drugs in the treatment of hypertension.** *Br Clin Pharmacol* 1982, **13**:51–60.

70. Solomon S, Hotchkiss E, Saravay SM, *et al.* **Impairment of memory function by antihypertensive medication.** *Arch Gen Psychiatry* 1983, **40**:1109–1112.

71. O'Malley K, Cox J, O'Brien E. **Choice of drug treatment for elderly hypertensive patients.** *Am J Med* 1991, **90** (suppl 3A):S27–S33.

72. Waal HJ. **Propranolol induced depression.** *Br Med J* 1967, **2**:50.

73. Burris JF. **β-blockers, dyslipidemia and coronary artery disease.** *Arch Intern Med* 1993, **153**:2085–2092.

74. Swainson CP, Winney RJ. **Effect of beta-blockade in chronic renal failure.** *Br Med J* 1976, **1**:459.

75. Yusuf S, Held P, Furberg C. **Update of effects of calcium antagonists in myocardial infarction or angina in light of the second Danish Verapamil Infarction Trial (DAVIT-II) and other recent studies.** *Am J Cardiol* 1991, **67**:1295–1297.

76. Gong L, Zhang W, Zhu Y, *et al.* **Shanghai Trial of Nifedipine in the Elderly (STONE).** *J Hypertens* 1996, **14**:1237–1245.

77. Leren P. **The cardiovascular effects of alpha-blocking agents.** *J Hypertens* 1992, **10** (suppl 3):S11–S15.

78. Anaszek WF, Kellerman D, Brogden RN, *et al.* **Prazosin – pharmacological properties and therapeutic use in hypertension and congestive heart failure.** *Drugs* 1983, **25**:339–384.

79. Guidelines Subcommittee. **1999 World Health Organization–International Society of Hypertension Guidelines for the Management of Hypertension.** *J Hypertens 1999*, **17**:151–183.

80. Joint National Committee on Prevention, Detection, Evaluation, and Treatment of High Bood Pressure. **The sixth report of the Joint National Committee on Prevention, Detection, Evaluation, and Treatment of High Bood Pressure.** *Arch Intern Med* 1997, **157**:2413–2446.

Index

COVERSYL® Abridged Prescribing Information.
(Refer to summary of Product Characteristics before prescribing). Coversyl (perindopril) Presentation: 2mg and 4mg tablets. Indications: Essential and Renovascular Hypertension. Congestive Heart Failure: In Congestive Heart Failure Coversyl should be used as adjunctive therapy with digitalis and/or diuretics. As with other ACE inhibitors, treatment with Coversyl should be initiated under close supervision. Dosage and Administration: Hypertension: 2mg once a day is the normal starting dose. Titrate dose to gain optimum blood pressure control. The usual maintenance dose is 4mg once daily. Maximum daily dose is 8mg once daily and may be combined with a diuretic. Coversyl should be taken before food. Congestive Heart Failure: Coversyl should be initiated under close supervision at a starting dose of 2mg taken in the morning which may be increased to 4mg (once blood pressure acceptability has been demonstrated). Diuretic-treated Patients: Stop the diuretic 3 days before starting Coversyl at 2mg. Diuretics can be re-started later if required, preferably at the lowest dose. Elderly: Start treatment under close supervision at 2mg daily. Impaired Renal Function: Coversyl should be used with caution adjusting the dose according to the creatinine clearance (see SPC). Children: Coversyl is not recommended. Contra-Indications: Patients with a history of hypersensitivity to Coversyl. Pregnancy - stop treatment if suspected. Women of child bearing potential - do not use unless protected with effective contraception. Lactation - not to be used in nursing mothers. Precautions: Assess renal function before and during treatment where appropriate. Hypotension may occur, particularly in those receiving diuretics or suffering from Congestive Heart Failure. However in comparative studies versus placebo and other ACE inhibitors, the first administration of 2mg of Coversyl to patients with mild to moderate heart failure was not associated with any significant reduction of blood pressure as compared to placebo. Renal Insufficiency, Renovascular Hypertension: renal function should be closely monitored. Surgery/Anaesthesia: hypotension may occur. Aortic stenosis/hypertrophic cardiomyopathy: use with caution. Interactions: Potassium supplements and potassium sparing diuretics are not recommended. Combination with antidiabetic agents may increase the hypoglycaemic effect. Combination with other antihypertensive agents, certain anaesthetics, neuroleptics or imipramine-type drugs may increase the hypotensive effect. Serum lithium concentrations may rise during lithium therapy. Side Effects: Cough, fatigue, asthenia, malaise, headache, disturbance of mood and/or sleep have been reported. Less often taste impairment, epigastric discomfort, nausea, abdominal pain, pruritus, flushing and rash. Reversible increases in blood urea and creatinine may be observed. Proteinuria has occurred in some patients. Rarely, angioneurotic oedema, neutropenia and decreases in haemoglobin, red cells and platelets have been reported. Basic NHS Cost: 2mg tablets, £9.45 for pack of 30. 4mg tablets, £13.65 for pack of 30. Legal Category: POM. Product Licence Numbers: 2mg tablets 5815/0001, 4mg tablets 5815/0002. Distributor: Servier Laboratories Ltd, Fulmer Hall, Windmill Road, Fulmer, Slough, SL3 6HH. Tel (01753) 662744. Coversyl® is a registered trademark.

Natrilix® SR 1.5mg Abridged Prescribing Information
(Please refer to summary of product characteristics before prescribing) Presentation: Sustained release coated tablets each containing 1.5mg indapamide. Uses: Essential hypertension. Dosage and Administration: Adults: The dosage is one tablet daily, preferably in the morning. Indapamide reduces left ventricular hypertrophy. It has been demonstrated that in the short, medium and long-term, in hypertensive patients, indapamide: • does not interfere with lipid metabolism: triglycerides, LDL-cholesterol and HDL cholesterol • does not interfere with carbohydrate metabolism, even in diabetic hypertensive patients. Contra-indications: hypersensitivity to sulphonamides: severe hepatic or renal impairment; hypokalaemia. Warnings, etc: In hepatic impairment, encephalopathy may occur; if so, stop Natrilix SR immediately. Plasma sodium should be measured before and at intervals during treatment. Plasma potassium should be monitored closely from the first week of treatment in patients in whom hypokalaemia presents a risk. Transitory rise in plasma calcium may occur. Gout attacks may increase in hyperuricaemic patients. Reduction in glomerular filtration due to hypovolaemia may worsen renal insufficiency. Interactions: The co-administration of Natrilix SR with lithium or drugs prolonging the QT interval or causing torsade de pointes is not recommended. Caution required in co-administration with NSAIDs, high dose salicylates, compounds causing hypokalaemia, baclofen or digitalis. Natrilix SR is not recommended in pregnancy or during breast feeding. Side effects: Hypokalaemia, hyponatraemia, hypovolaemia, increased plasma uric acid and blood glucose, very rarely - haematological events, hypercalcaemia. Hypersensitivity reactions, skin rashes, worsening of acute disseminated lupus erythematosis. Rarely, nausea, constipation, dry mouth, vertigo, fatigue, paraesthesia, headache. Very rarely, pancreatitis. Basic NHS Cost: 30 tabs £4.47. Marketing Authorisation Number: PL05815/0010. Legal Category: POM. Full prescribing information is available on request from: Servier Laboratories Ltd., Fulmer Hall, Windmill Road, Fulmer, Slough SL3 6HH. Tel (01753) 666228. Date of preparation: June 1999.